EVERYTHING ABOUT

FRUITARIAN DIET

Complete Nutritional Cookbook, Foods, Meal Plan And Recipes To Nourishing the Body, Satisfying the Soul and Discovering the Wholeness of Living

DR. ALVIN BRANTLEY

© 2023 ALVIN BRANTLEY

All rights reserved. No part of this book may be reproduced, stored, or transmitted in any form or by any means, electronic, mechanical, photocopying, recording, scanning, or otherwise, without the prior written permission of the author.

Disclaimer

The information provided in this book is intended for general informational purposes only. It is not a substitute for professional medical advice, diagnosis, or treatment.

You should not use the information in this book for diagnosing or treating a health problem or disease by self decision. Always seek the advice of your physician or other qualified health provider with any questions you may have regarding a medical condition.

The author and publisher of this book make no representations or warranties with respect to the accuracy, applicability, fitness, or completeness of the contents of this book. The information contained in this book is based on the author's research and experience, and it is shared with the understanding that the author is not engaged in rendering medical, health, or any other kind of professional advice for you by this book.

The author does not endorse or promote any specific products, brands, or companies related to the contents provided in this book.

Any mention of products or services in this book is for informational purposes only and does not constitute an endorsement.

The author has not entered into any affiliate marketing agreements and has not signed any endorsement deals with individuals, organizations, or companies.

Readers are encouraged to consult with their healthcare providers before making any dietary or lifestyle chaSnges based on the information provided in this book. The author and publisher disclaim any liability for the decisions made by readers based on the information in this book.

Contents

CHAPTER ONE...................................12

A Fruitarian Diet: What Is It?..............12

A Synopsis Of Fruitarian Lifestyle History...................................12

Advantages Of A Fruitarian Diet 13

Obstacles In A Fruitarian Diet.........14

CHAPTER TWO....................................16

Compassion For Fruitarianism............16

The Theory Underpinning Fruitarianism 17

Fundamentals Of A Fruitarian Diet .18

Differentiating This Plant-Based Diet From Others 20

CHAPTER THREE 22

Healthy Foundations...........................22

Fruits' Essential Nutrients 22

Fulfilling Daily Nutritional Needs....23

Possible Nutritional Shortfalls And Solutions 24

CHAPTER FOUR 26

Centers Of The Fruitarian Diet 26

Variety Of Fruits 26

Various Fruit Types 27

Local And Seasonal Fruits................28

Unique Fruits And Their Advantages 28

CHAPTER FIVE...............................32

Meal Recipes And Planning 32

Examples Of Menus..........................33

Delectable Recipes For Fruitarians..34

Advantages Of A Fruitarian Diet......35

Obstacles And Things To Think About 35

CHAPTER SIX 38

Agriculture And Health......................38

Effects On Human Health................38

Emotional And Mental Health 39

Fruitarian Diet And Lifespan 40

Typical Problems And Their Fixes: ..42

Handling Nutritional Issues: 43

Overcoming Potential Drawbacks: ..44

CHAPTER SEVEN 46

Fruitarianism In Various Livelihoods.46

Fruitarianism In Sportsmen 46

Family-Friendly Fruitarianism 47

Traveling And Fruitarianism 48

Discussions Among The Community Of Firefighters 49

Consumption Of Fruits In Media 51

CHAPTER EIGHT 54

Changing To A Fruitarian Mode Of Life 54

Transitioning Gradually Vs. Immediately.......................................54

Advice For A Seamless Changeover .56

Looking For Expert Advice 57

Conclusion 58

Considering The Fruitarian Path 59

Progressing: Enduring Fruitarianism 60

Introduction

The Fruitarian Diet is a novel dietary strategy that emphasizes fruit consumption, however, some versions permit the addition of nuts, seeds, and specific plant-based meals as well. Proponents of this way of living claim that eating mostly fruits provides several health advantages and is in line with human nature.

This dietary philosophy is based on the notion that eating foods in their purest form—especially fruits—promotes optimal health.

CHAPTER ONE

A Fruitarian Diet: What Is It?

The intake of raw fruits is the fundamental component of the fruitarian diet. This covers a wide range of fruits, including citrus fruits, apples, bananas, berries, and more. Nuts, seeds, and delicate, leafy greens may also be allowed in some Fruitarian Diet versions.

The diet places a strong emphasis on eating entire, unprocessed foods as they are; cooking and other food-processing methods are discouraged.

A Synopsis Of Fruitarian Lifestyle History

The Fruitarian Diet has its origins in early human history, as evidenced by references to diets centered on fruits found in many different cultures. Because they were closely connected to nature, some ancient societies adopted fruitarianism as a means of balancing with their surroundings.

The Fruitarian Diet became well-known in the modern era as a component of the larger raw food movement that surfaced in the late 19th and early 20th century. Prominent figures in this movement, such as Ann Wigmore and Maximilian Bircher-Brenner, promoted the advantages of eating raw, unprocessed foods, such as fruits.

Advantages Of A Fruitarian Diet

Advocates of the Fruitarian Diet assert that this way of living has numerous health advantages. Fruits' high vitamin, mineral, antioxidant, and fiber content is thought to promote general health. Proponents of the fruitarian diet claim that it can improve digestion, boost energy levels, and improve mental clarity. The diet is also frequently commended for its possible assistance in controlling weight and preventing several chronic illnesses.

Obstacles In A Fruitarian Diet

The Fruitarian Diet has many potential advantages, but it is not without difficulties. Meeting nutritional demands is one major challenge, since a diet high in fruits may be deficient in several critical nutrients.

A few nutrients that could need extra care are protein, calcium, vitamin B12, and omega-3 fatty acids. Also, for those who adhere to the Fruitarian Diet, finding a wide variety of year-round, high-quality fruits and handling certain digestive problems, including bloating or diarrhea, can be difficult.

To guarantee a well-rounded and balanced dietary intake, practitioners must approach this lifestyle with much thought and may even consult with nutritionists or healthcare providers for advice.

CHAPTER TWO

Compassion For Fruitarianism

A fruitarian diet focuses on eating only fruits, seeds, nuts, and other plant-based foods that can be harvested without causing harm to the plants. This distinctive dietary strategy has its roots in a philosophy that takes ethical, environmental, and spiritual factors into account in addition to nutrition. Fruitarianism emphasizes a deep relationship with the plant kingdom and offers a unique approach to feeding the body and engaging with nature.

The Theory Underpinning Fruitarianism

Fruitarianism is based on a deep regard for the natural world and all living things. Proponents of this way of life think that eating available foods without harming the plant or its ability to reproduce is a good idea. Fruitarianism's ethical foundation frequently includes considerations for the environmental effects of dietary decisions.

Some fruitarians follow this route to reduce their environmental impact and make food decisions that are more in line with a larger sustainable philosophy.

For some practitioners, the ideology even has a spiritual component, seeing eating fruits and plant-based meals as a means of achieving a closer relationship with nature. For many, fruitarianism is a way of life that embodies a profound understanding of the interdependence of all living things rather than just a diet. This spiritual viewpoint frequently incorporates the idea that plant-based meals have life force and energy that promote general well-being.

Fundamentals Of A Fruitarian Diet

Fruits are the main item consumed on a fruitarian diet; additional foods derived from plants, such as seeds and nuts, are also included. The main idea is to emphasize a diet that supports plants in their natural lifespan by consuming items that can be obtained without harming the plant. A broad variety of fresh, ripe fruits are usually served with fruitarian meals, highlighting the diversity found in nature. For variation and extra nutritional value, some practitioners also include nuts and seeds.

The Fruitarian Diet places a strong focus on unprocessed and raw foods. To maintain the nutritional value and enzymes of fruits and vegetables, many fruitarians recommend eating them raw. This is consistent with the idea that heating these items could deplete their energy and life force. Within the Fruitarian group, however, there are differences in individual preferences; some may include a small quantity of cooked or processed food in their diet.

Differentiating This Plant-Based Diet From Others

Although there are many similarities between fruitarianism and other plant-based diets, such as veganism and vegetarianism, it differs in that it places particular emphasis on fruits and plant-based meals that may be gathered without causing harm to the plant.

Fruitarian meals mostly consist of fresh, whole, unprocessed fruits, in contrast to certain plant-based diets that incorporate grains, legumes, and processed foods. This distinction emphasizes the dedication to a diet that emphasizes foods in their purest, most natural form, reflecting the ethical and ecological issues that are central to Fruitarian philosophy.

Fruitarianism is a holistic lifestyle that integrates ethical, environmental, and spiritual concerns beyond just dietary choices.

The main tenets of the diet are to consume plant-based foods in a way that minimizes harm to living things and respects the natural lifetime of plants. As fruitarianism becomes more popular, it presents a distinctive viewpoint on conscious and sustainable living through dietary decisions.

CHAPTER THREE

Healthy Foundations

The Fruitarian Diet is a dietary approach that focuses primarily on consuming fruits in all of their forms. Its foundation is fruit consumption. Proponents of this diet contend that people can obtain the vital nutrients, vitamins, and minerals required for optimum health by eating solely fruits. To evaluate the possible advantages and disadvantages of the fruitarian diet, it is critical to comprehend its nutritional underpinnings.

Fruits' Essential Nutrients

Fruits are well known for having a high content of key nutrients that are necessary for human health. They usually include a variety of vitamins, such as potassium, folate, and vitamin C. In addition, fruits include a substantial amount of dietary fiber, which supports satiety and improves digestive health. Fruit antioxidants including flavonoids and carotenoids are essential in the fight against oxidative stress. Examining the range of vital nutrients found in fruits can shed light on the possible health advantages of a fruitarian diet.

Fulfilling Daily Nutritional Needs

A fruitarian diet should take into account several factors, one of which is how well it will fulfill daily nutritional needs. Fruits are rich in nutrients, but some may be less abundant than others, so careful dietary planning is necessary. For instance, it can be difficult to consume enough protein and necessary fatty acids from fruits alone. As a result, to meet their daily nutritional requirements, those who follow this diet need to deliberately vary the fruits they choose.

Possible Nutritional Shortfalls And Solutions

Even though fruits have a high nutrient content, those following a fruitarian diet may still have some nutritional deficits. Fruits often have lower protein content than other food groups, so protein insufficiency is a regular worry. Incorporating fruits high in protein, such as guava and kiwi, or adding plant-based protein sources could help close this gap. Furthermore, consideration should be given to consuming important fatty acids, such as omega-3s, through the inclusion of particular foods or appropriate supplements.

The Fruitarian Diet offers a distinctive approach to nutrition because of its emphasis on fruit consumption.

A fruitarian diet must be effectively adopted and maintained, and key components include comprehending the nutritional underpinnings, recognizing vital nutrients in fruits, and filling in any nutritional shortfalls. Those who are thinking about adopting this dietary practice should make educated decisions and, if needed, consult medical professionals to guarantee a sustainable and well-rounded approach to nutrition.

CHAPTER FOUR

Centers Of The Fruitarian Diet

centered on fruit-eating, with followers avoiding all other food groups from their diet. This diet plan is predicated on the idea that eating only fruits is in line with what people naturally eat. We examine the several kinds of fruits that are the cornerstone of the fruitarian diet in our investigation of this eating style.

Variety Of Fruits

Fruits are available in many different varieties, each with its special blend of nutrients, flavors, and textures. The Fruitarian Diet promotes the intake of a wide variety of fruits, from the more exotic dragon fruit and persimmons to the more commonplace apples and bananas. This kind guarantees a wider range of vital vitamins and minerals in addition to adding to the gastronomic pleasure.

Various Fruit Types

The Fruitarian Diet places a strong focus on accepting a wide variety of fruit types. Berries, citrus fruits, tropical fruits, stone fruits, and melons are examples of this, but they're not the only ones.

The justification for this variety stems from the idea that various fruits have unique nutritional advantages, and by including a wide range, people can get a more complete range of vital elem

Local And Seasonal Fruits

The intake of fruits that are in season and locally sourced is frequently given priority by followers of the fruitarian diet.

This method supports the theory that fruits that are in season are more in line with the body's natural requirements during particular periods of the year. Selecting fruits that grow nearby is also seen as a sustainable strategy that boosts local agriculture and lessens the environmental effect of long-distance driving.

Unique Fruits And Their Advantages

Exotic fruits, which are frequently not indigenous to the person adhering to the diet, are also accepted in the Fruitarian

Diet. The exotic fruits durian, lychee, passion fruit, and jackfruit are a few examples.

Proponents contend that including these exotic fruits broadens the variety of flavors and nutrients available, enlivening the diet and possibly providing special health advantages.

Fruitarian diet proponents claim that because fruits are high in vitamins, minerals, fiber, and antioxidants, they can provide all of the body's nutritional needs.

Critics counter that this diet can be deficient in important elements including fat, protein, and several vitamins and minerals that are present in other food groups.

People thinking about going on a fruitarian diet should speak with medical professionals as with any restrictive diet to make sure their nutritional needs are satisfied and any potential deficiencies are taken care of.

CHAPTER FIVE

Meal Recipes And Planning

Making Well-Composed Fruitarian Meals

Planning meals is essential while following a fruitarian diet to guarantee a balanced intake of nutrients.

The nutritious composition of fruits varies greatly, therefore it's important to pay close attention to the macronutrients, vitamins, and minerals that are necessary. Generally speaking, a fruitarian meal consists of a range of fruits that provide a spectrum of nutrients. Fruits with varying textures, flavors, and colors should be combined to create a varied nutritional profile.

A fruitarian meal plan must carefully take dietary requirements and tastes into account. When following a fruitarian diet, a person may eat a range of fruits throughout the day to maintain a healthy balance of fats, proteins, and carbohydrates.

One might have a smoothie for breakfast consisting of frozen berries, bananas, and a small amount of almonds.

A vibrant fruit salad made with a combination of tropical and regional fruits could be served for lunch. Dinner may be something heavier, like an avocado and raw veggie and fruit wrap.

Delectable Recipes For Fruitarians

The Fruitarian Diet inspires people to experiment with a variety of delectable foods by fostering their creativity in the kitchen.

The options are endless and intriguing, ranging from exotic fruit smoothie bowls to cool fruit salads. Seasonal fruits are frequently used in fruitarian cuisine, creating a delicious fusion of textures and flavors. Mango and pineapple salsa, watermelon, and mint salad, and banana-based ice cream are a few of the well-liked recipes.

These recipes satisfy Fruitarianism's dietary requirements while also pleasing the palate with their inherent freshness and sweetness.

Advantages Of A Fruitarian Diet

Proponents of the Fruitarian Diet point out several possible advantages of this eating pattern. Fruits' high fiber content aids in digestive health and their wealth of vitamins and minerals promote general well-being.

Antioxidants, which are abundant in fruits, are essential in preventing oxidative stress and lowering inflammation. The Fruitarian Diet is also commended for its simplicity in encouraging a sustainable and low-key way of eating.

Obstacles And Things To Think About

The Fruitarian Diet has many health advantages, but there are drawbacks and things to think about as well. The possibility of nutritional shortages is one major issue, especially about vitamin B12, iron, calcium, and omega-3 fatty acids. Fruitarianism may need to fill these nutritional shortfalls by careful planning or supplementation.

The cost and accessibility of a wide variety of fresh fruits is another factor to take into account, which may be restricted for people residing in particular areas.

The Fruitarian Diet is a lifestyle choice that emphasizes eating only fresh fruits. It offers a distinctive perspective on health and nutrition.

People who are thinking about adopting this diet should be aware of the difficulties and dietary requirements even though it may have health benefits. Organizing meals is essential to consuming a varied and well-balanced diet, and trying out delectable Fruitarian recipes brings a fun element to this way of eating.

In the end, implementing a fruitarian diet calls for thoughtful thought and customized preparation to accommodate each person's unique dietary requirements and preferences.

CHAPTER SIX

Agriculture And Health

Fruitarianism is a diet philosophy that emphasizes eating mostly raw and uncooked foods. It centers on the consumption of fruits, seeds, nuts, and some plants.

Fruitarian diet proponents think that eating this way can improve general health and well-being. However, there are concerns over this dietary approach's effects on mental and emotional health, physical health, and even longevity.

Effects On Human Health

Fresh fruit consumption is the main focus of the fruitarian diet because it is high in vital vitamins, minerals, and antioxidants.

Advocates contend that by giving the body the resources it needs for optimum operation, this nutrient-dense diet may promote physical health. Critics, however, point out that a diet centered only on fruits may leave one deficient in many important nutrients, especially protein, calcium, and vitamin B12. Maintaining general physical health still depends on finding a balance and making sure you're getting a varied supply of nutrients.

Emotional And Mental Health

Fruitarians frequently assert that the diet has a favorable impact on mental and emotional health in addition to physical health. Eating nutrient-dense fruits is thought to improve brain clarity and promote cognitive function. Furthermore, some people claim that adopting a fruitarian lifestyle improves their emotional stability and mood. The psychological effects of following such a rigid diet are not without difficulties, though. Critics contend that the necessity for careful meal planning and the possibility of social isolation could have a detrimental effect on mental and emotional well-being.

Fruitarian Diet And Lifespan

Fruitarianism's supposed link to a long life is one of its fascinating features. Proponents of the theory contend that fruits' high antioxidant content may have an anti-aging impact and lengthen longevity. Though studies on the health advantages of eating fruits and vegetables are well-established, there is little scientific evidence explicitly connecting a fruitarian diet to longer lifespans. However, as genetics, lifestyle choices, and individual characteristics all have a substantial impact on life expectancy, it is imperative to proceed with caution when interpreting claims of longevity.

Making the switch to a fruitarian diet presents significant questions about its effects on longevity, mental and emotional health, and physical health. Although the diet is rich in vital nutrients, its limited nature necessitates close monitoring to guarantee adequate intake of these nutrients.

To fully comprehend fruitarianism's long-term impacts and their ramifications for general health and lifespan, more research is required.

Typical Problems And Their Fixes: Handling Social circumstances: Handling social circumstances where dietary preferences could conflict with traditional norms is one of the major obstacles experienced by persons who adhere to the Fruitarian Diet. Finding appropriate options at social gatherings or activities that revolve around food might be difficult for Fruitarians.

Planning and efficient communication are often key components of solutions to this problem. Notifying guests ahead of time about dietary requirements enables accommodations, and sharing fruit-based dishes can promote tolerance and acceptance.

Handling Nutritional Issues:
Following a fruitarian diet may lead to a reduction in some important nutrients, which can raise nutritional issues. Although fruits are often high in vitamins and minerals, it is possible to have inadequacies in calcium, vitamin B12, and protein. Fruitarians must carefully arrange their diet to include a range of fruits, nuts, and seeds to allay these worries and provide a balanced intake of vital nutrients. To satisfy certain nutritional needs, supplements or foods fortified with ingredients may also be taken into consideration.

Overcoming Potential Drawbacks:
Although the fruitarian diet has advantages, there may also be disadvantages that people should be aware of and take into consideration. Because fruits contain a lot of fiber, some people may have digestive problems that cause bloating or discomfort.

Fruitarians must pay close attention to their bodies and incorporate these foods into their diets gradually. Concerns over energy levels and calorie intake may also surface.

To guarantee a fruitarian lifestyle that is both sustainable and beneficial, it can be helpful to monitor nutritional intake and seek advice from a healthcare practitioner.

The Fruitarian Diet has drawbacks that need to be carefully considered in addition to the potential for enhanced health and wellbeing.

To successfully adopt and sustain a Fruitarian lifestyle, effective communication, dietary planning, and awareness of potential downsides are critical components.

CHAPTER SEVEN

Fruitarianism In Various Livelihoods

Consuming fruits, seeds, nuts, and other plant-based foods that can be gathered without causing harm to the plant is the main component of the fruitarian diet. Emphasizing a diet centered around ripe and fresh fruits, it is frequently seen as a subset of veganism.

This lifestyle option has grown in favor among a variety of groups, fitting in with distinct advantages and considerations for varied lives.

Fruitarianism In Sportsmen

Strict diet plans are frequently followed by athletes to maximize their performance and general well-being. Fruitarianism has gained popularity among certain sportsmen due to its emphasis on natural energy sources and fresh fruits.

Vital elements from the diet—such as vitamins, minerals, and antioxidants—can support better healing and long-term energy levels.

On the other hand, athletes who switch to a fruitarian diet must carefully organize their meals to make sure they get enough protein and energy.

Family-Friendly Fruitarianism

Families who are considering fruitarianism as a dietary option must address the dietary requirements of people of different ages.

Even though a fruitarian diet can be very high in vital nutrients, parents still need to make sure that their kids get enough of the vitamins, minerals, and proteins that are necessary for healthy growth and development.

Families adopting fruitarianism must prioritize education and thoughtful meal preparation to thrive as a unit while satisfying each member's nutritional needs.

Traveling And Fruitarianism

The peripatetic lifestyle might offer advantages and disadvantages to those following a fruitarian diet. Positively, fruitarians can sample a variety of gastronomic pleasures since many locations provide an abundance of fresh and exotic fruits.

 Obstacles could include finding fruits readily available and finding a balanced diet when traveling.

For fruitarian travelers to make sure they adhere to their dietary beliefs without sacrificing nutrients when traveling, preparation, research, and adaptability are essential.

Discussions Among The Community Of Firefighters

The ideal food composition is a topic of continuous discussion among the Fruitarian community. While some devotees just eat fruits, others might also eat nuts, seeds, and specific veggies. The argument also revolves around the proper ratio of raw to cooked meals.

While some Fruitarians support a strictly raw diet, others believe that it is beneficial to include some gently cooked foods for flavor and diversity.

There are also disagreements on whether a fruitarian lifestyle is sustainable over the long run.

While some people claim to have thrived on this diet for extended periods, others voice worries about possible long-term health problems. These discussions highlight the significance of individualized strategies to address dietary demands and the individual variety in how people may react to the fruitarian diet.

Consumption Of Fruits In Media

The fruitarian diet has drawn interest from mainstream and alternative media sources alike. Some present it as a drastic and maybe dangerous dietary option, while others feature success stories of people who report increased vitality and health. Fruitarianism-related sentiments are further polarized by the media's tendency to highlight extreme situations. It is necessary to assess media representations critically and take into account a range of Fruitarian experiences.

The Fruitarian diet is a unique nutritional philosophy that has its ardent proponents and detractors. knowing Fruitarianism's intricacies requires addressing common objections, managing internal arguments, and knowing how the religion is portrayed in the media.

Like with any dietary decision, what works for one person may not work for another. This is why it is important to consider individual considerations, nutritional planning, and a comprehensive understanding of the advantages and disadvantages of the diet.

CHAPTER EIGHT

Changing To A Fruitarian Mode Of Life

A fruitarian diet emphasizes eating fruits as the main source of nutrition, which represents a significant change in eating habits. The focus of this diet is on eating raw fruits only—along with seeds and nuts—while avoiding grains, processed foods, and animal products. A balanced and nutritionally sufficient diet must be ensured while making the switch to a fruitarian lifestyle, which calls for considerable thought and preparation.

Transitioning Gradually Vs. Immediately

Deciding to go to a Fruitarian lifestyle gradually or all at once is one of the most important ones that people think about it have to make. A progressive transition entails phasing out other food groups and gradually adding more fruits to the diet. This approach is frequently preferred since it lowers the risk of nutritional shortages and digestive distress by allowing the body to adjust to the changes gradually.

Conversely, individuals may choose to make a sudden change, suddenly cutting out non-fruit foods from their diet. This method may result in quicker adaption, but it may also present problems including signs of detoxification and possible nutritional imbalances.

Advice For A Seamless Changeover

Adopting a Fruitarian lifestyle requires careful attention to many areas of one's food and lifestyle, regardless of the transition method used.

It is crucial to make sure you are getting enough of the important nutrients, such as proteins, minerals, and vitamins.

The danger of vitamin shortages can be reduced by consuming a variety of fruits. A wide range of nutrients is also ensured by including fruits of different hues and varieties.

Because fruits contain a lot of water, people following a fruitarian diet should be mindful of how much fluid they consume. During the shift, consulting reliable sources of knowledge and making connections with seasoned professionals can offer insightful advice.

Looking For Expert Advice

Making the switch to a fruitarian diet requires negotiating various obstacles, and getting expert advice can help to ensure a successful and long-lasting change. Dietitians or nutritionists with experience in plant-based diets can provide individualized guidance by accounting for lifestyle variables, nutritional requirements, and specific medical concerns.

These experts may assist in creating a Fruitarian diet plan that is well-balanced, address worries about possible nutrient deficiencies, and, if needed, offer advice on supplements. Frequent check-ins with a medical professional can also aid in keeping an eye on general health and addressing any new problems. Professional assistance is especially important for people who may be more vulnerable to nutrient imbalances or have pre-existing medical issues. In general, consulting with medical specialists increases the chances of a seamless and health-conscious switch to a Fruitarian way of life.

Conclusion

To sum up, the Fruitarian diet is a distinct approach to nutrition that places a focus on consuming raw, fresh fruits. Critics point to practical difficulties and dietary deficits, while supporters emphasize possible health benefits and a link to nature. It is necessary to weigh both viewpoints fairly when reflecting on the Fruitarian path, keeping in mind personal health requirements and lifestyle choices.

Considering The Fruitarian Path

Thinking back on the Fruitarian experience entails evaluating for oneself the advantages and difficulties encountered when following this dietary philosophy.

People might think about adjustments to their general health, intestinal health, and energy levels. People can use this introspective process to help them decide whether a fruitarian diet is right for them and their particular needs.

Progressing: Enduring Fruitarianism

The idea of sustainable Fruitarianism becomes essential as people travel the Fruitarian path. This entails striking a balance between the diet's tenets and real-world factors that affect long-term compliance.

A variety of fruits, nutritional supplements, and diet modifications based on personal preferences and medical needs are all possible components of sustainable fruitarianism. Striking this balance is vital for those determined to embrace Fruitarianism as a lasting and meaningful lifestyle choice.

www.ingramcontent.com/pod-product-compliance
Lightning Source LLC
Chambersburg PA
CBHW060808260726
48660CB00002B/832